Background

The Patient Protection and Affordable Care Act of 2010[1] and the Health Care and Education Reconciliation Act of 2010[2] (collectively referred to as the Affordable Care Act) were signed into law in March 2010. Together they contain more than 500 provisions intended to make health insurance more affordable and available to individuals. The Affordable Care Act will impact every aspect of health care for individuals, employers, insurers, hospitals and medical personnel, health and tax practitioners, health advocacy groups, and other health providers. Revenue provisions contained in the legislation are designed to generate $438 billion to help pay for the overall cost of health care reform.[3]

More than 40 of the 500 provisions added to or amended the Internal Revenue Code. The tax provisions provide incentives and tax breaks to individuals and small businesses to offset health care expenses. They also impose penalties for individuals and businesses that do not obtain health care coverage for themselves or their employees. For example, one provision of the Affordable Care Act is the requirement for individuals to maintain minimum essential health care coverage or face a continuous penalty. The penalty will be imposed on any taxpayer who, for any month after Calendar Year 2013, fails to maintain minimum essential health care coverage.[4]

The Affordable Care Act establishes new reporting requirements for employers and health insurance providers

The Affordable Care Act includes provisions that establish new information return reporting and sharing requirements for third parties (*e.g.*, employers and health insurers) and the Health Insurance Exchanges (the Exchanges). The reported information will be used to administer the Advance Premium Tax Credit,[5] the individual mandate to obtain health insurance, and the employer minimum essential coverage requirement. The Internal Revenue Service (IRS) has also been given the authority to share certain tax data with other Federal and State agencies to be used to determine eligibility for the Advance Premium Tax Credit. Implementing these reporting provisions will require the IRS to engage external stakeholders, develop internal and external

---

[1] Pub. L. No. 111-148, 124 Stat. 119 (2010) (codified as amended in scattered sections of the U.S. Code), as amended by the Health Care and Education Reconciliation Act of 2010, Pub. L. No. 111-152, 124 Stat. 1029 (2010).
[2] Pub. L. No. 111-152, 124 Stat. 1029 (2010).
[3] Joint Committee on Taxation, JCX-17-10, Estimated Revenue Effects of the Amendment in the Nature of a Substitute to H.R. 4872, the "Reconciliation Act of 2010," as Amended, in Combination With the Revenue Effects of H.R. 3590, the "Patient Protection and Affordable Care Act ('PPACA')," as Passed by the Senate, and Scheduled for Consideration by the House Committee on Rules on March 20, 2010 (Mar. 20, 2010).
[4] See Appendix IV for a glossary of terms.
[5] The Advance Premium Tax Credit subsidizes the purchase of certain health insurance plans obtained through an Exchange. The credit is refundable and payable in advance directly to the insurer.

education and outreach initiatives, develop formal and informal guidance including forms and publications, and develop systems and processes to receive and use the information provided. Figure 1 identifies these key information reporting provisions.

Figure 1: Key Affordable Care Act Information Reporting Provisions

Provision	Effective Date of the Reporting Requirements	Details
1502: Reporting of Health Insurance Coverage (Internal Revenue Code Section 6055).	Businesses and individuals are required to file a health insurance report for Calendar Year 2014 in January 2015.	Requires that every business and individual who provides "minimum essential coverage" to any individual during a calendar year report to the IRS certain health insurance information. This information includes the names of the individuals obtaining health coverage, the dates of health coverage, and whether the coverage is a qualified health plan offered through an Exchange.
1514: Reporting of Employer Health Insurance Coverage (Internal Revenue Code Section 6056).	Large employers are required to report on the availability of minimum essential coverage during Calendar Year 2014 in January 2015.	Requires large employers (average 50 full-time equivalent employees in the preceding calendar year) to file an information return with the IRS to report whether they offer their employees and their dependents the opportunity to enroll in minimum essential health care coverage, the period an employee must wait to become enrolled, and information regarding those employees who are enrolled in such coverage. The employers must also provide full-time employees a copy of the information returns they provide to the IRS.
9002: Inclusion of Employer Health Coverage on Form W-2, *Wage and Tax Statement* (Internal Revenue Code Section 6051).	Large employers are required to report for Calendar Year 2012 on Forms W-2 distributed in January 2013. Employers that are not considered large employers are not required to report prior to January 2014.	Requires large employers to report the total dollar value of health insurance coverage sponsored by the employer on each employee's annual Form W-2. Although this information is included on the Form W-2, the amount reported is not counted as taxable income.
9010: Imposition of Annual Fee on Health Insurance Providers.	Health insurance providers are required to file a net premiums report for Calendar Year 2013 in May 2014.	Imposes an annual fee on health insurance providers whose net premiums written during the calendar year exceed $25 million. The annual fee requirement will begin no later than September 30, 2014. Each insurance provider is responsible for filing a premiums report with the IRS. Failure to file the report will generally result in an assessed penalty of $10,000 plus the lesser of $1,000 times the number of days the report is not filed timely or the amount of the fee required to be paid by the health insurance provider.

Source: Affordable Care Act.

This review was performed in the IRS's Affordable Care Act Office in Washington, D.C., during the period August through December 2012. We conducted this performance audit in accordance with generally accepted government auditing standards. Those standards require that we plan and perform the audit to obtain sufficient, appropriate evidence to provide a reasonable basis for our findings and conclusions based on our audit objective. We believe that the evidence obtained provides a reasonable basis for our findings and conclusions based on our audit objective. Detailed information on our audit objective, scope, and methodology is presented in Appendix I. Major contributors to the report are listed in Appendix II.

Results of Review

Implementation of Information Reporting Is Progressing; However, Improvements Are Needed to Ensure Compliance With Affordable Care Act Provisions

In June 2012, the Treasury Inspector General for Tax Administration (TIGTA) reported that the IRS had developed appropriate plans to implement key Affordable Care Act reporting provisions.[6] These plans address the development of tax forms, instructions, and publications; employee training; outreach and guidance to taxpayers and preparers; and computer programming and data needs. During this review, we determined that the IRS has continued to make progress in implementing the information reporting requirements relating to Affordable Care Act Provisions 1502, 1514, 9002, and 9010.

However, the implementation plan for Provision 9002 does not address how the IRS will ensure employer compliance with the reporting requirement. Additional third-party information could expand the IRS's ability to ensure taxpayer compliance with the Affordable Care Act provisions and requirements.

Implementing Affordable Care Act information reporting requirements is progressing

Since June 2012, the IRS has continued its efforts to ensure that it is ready to implement Affordable Care Act Provisions 1502, 1514, 9002, and 9010 by:

- Updating Form W-2 to include a box for employers to report the total dollar value of health insurance coverage provided to an employee. The form and related instructions for preparing the form were also updated and posted to the IRS website (www.IRS.gov).

- Identifying the information employers and insurers are required to provide for each of the provisions and developing draft tax forms that will be used to report this information to the IRS. The IRS also implemented two tiers of review for each of the draft tax forms developed. The first level of review, conducted by the Tax Forms and Publications function, identifies the forms, publications, and instructions that need to be revised to fulfill the legislative requirements. The second level of review is the business assessment

---

[6] TIGTA, Ref. No. 2012-43-064, *Affordable Care Act: Planning Efforts for the Tax Provisions of the Patient Protection and Affordable Care Act Appear Adequate; However, the Resource Estimation Process Needs Improvement* (June 2012).

completed by subject matter experts in the business area aided by the Tax Forms and Publications function.

- Developing processes to receive information required to be reported by employers and insurers. For example, the IRS developed processes to successfully receive the revised Forms W-2 from 18,513 large employers required to report the total dollar value of health insurance coverage provided to the individuals they employ on their Forms W-2.

- Developing and administering outreach and educational initiatives to provide information relating to these provisions to outside stakeholders. For example, the IRS provided an IRS webinar and developed a YouTube video on *Reporting of Employer Health Care Coverage on Form W-2*. The IRS plans to provide similar information for the other provisions using PowerPoint presentations, YouTube videos, and webinars.

- Developing training and additional guidance for IRS employees on the information reporting requirements relating to these provisions. For example, the IRS plans to develop and conduct training for IRS employees on these new provisions, including how to assist employers and insurers in complying with the reporting guidelines.

In addition, the IRS has identified the information system support needed to receive the information reported by employers and insurers, and it is in the process of developing the computer systems necessary to process and use this information.

The time frame for implementing Provision 9010 increases the risk of incorrectly computing annual fees

Our review identified concerns regarding the time frames the IRS has established for implementing Provision 9010. Provision 9010 imposes an annual fee on health insurance providers whose net premiums written during the calendar year exceed $25 million. The IRS is required to apportion $8 billion in annual fees among all health insurance providers whose net premiums for health insurance policies issued during Calendar Year 2013 exceed $25 million. The amount of the annual fee for each insurer is determined based on a ratio of the insurer's net premiums written compared to total net premiums of all insurers written during the previous calendar year. The annual fee requirement will begin no later than September 30, 2014.

The IRS will use the information returns required by Provision 9010 to apportion the $8 billion. The IRS does not plan to require health insurance providers to file these information returns until May 1, 2014, and does not plan to notify the insurers of the preliminary calculation of the annual fee until June 15, 2014. It plans to mail notices for the final annual fee calculation to insurers no later than August 31, 2014.

This timeline allows the IRS only four months to process preliminary fee determinations and any corrections to collect the $8 billion in fees for Fiscal Year 2014. The IRS is aware of the risk of incorrect annual fee assessments created by the compressed planned implementation timeline. However, the IRS responded that it must balance the need to provide health insurance providers adequate time to comply with the reporting requirement with the need to provide insurers adequate time to pay the annual fee by September 30, 2014. IRS management believes their implementation timeline will provide the balance needed and is taking steps to develop processes to timely verify that all health insurance providers have filed an information return as required. We plan to perform a subsequent review of the implementation of Provision 9010 as part of our continued audit coverage of the Affordable Care Act.

The implementation plan for Provision 9002 does not include the actions the IRS plans to take to ensure that large employers comply with reporting requirements

Most of the implementation plans appropriately address the processes needed to receive and use Affordable Care Act reporting information and include the steps needed to identify noncompliance with the provisions. Figure 2 shows the results of our analysis of the IRS's plans and whether the plans include actions to receive and use information and monitor compliance with the respective provision.

Figure 2: Evaluation of the IRS's Plans to Receive and Use Information and Monitor Compliance With Provisions

Provision	Plan Addresses Development of Processes Needed to Receive Information	Plan Addresses How the Information Received Will Be Used	Plan Addresses Steps to Be Taken to Identify Noncompliance
1502	✓	✓	✓
1514	✓	✓	✓
9002	✓	X	X
9010	✓	✓	✓

Source: TIGTA analysis of IRS planning documents for Affordable Care Act Provisions 1502, 1514, 9002, and 9010.

Only the plan for Provision 9002 excludes how the IRS will use the information being reported or how it will ensure that large employers comply with the law. The IRS acknowledges that there is a risk employers may miscalculate the cost of health care or simply not report the information required under Provision 9002. Nevertheless, the implementation plan does not include steps to ensure that employers report the information as required or to ensure that the information reported on Forms W-2 is accurate. Without this information, the IRS reduces its ability to verify eligibility compliance with other Affordable Care Act provisions. For example, the IRS can use the information reported on Forms W-2 to verify individuals' compliance with the individual health insurance mandate. In addition, information reported on Forms W-2 can also be used to identify individuals not eligible for the Premium Tax Credit because the individual has employer-paid health care coverage.

IRS management indicated that the information reported on Forms W-2 is solely for the purpose of providing consumer awareness. As such, the IRS does not consider reporting compliance for this provision as a high priority. Because the reporting was optional for all employers for Calendar Year 2011 and remains so for many employers for Calendar Year 2012, IRS management indicated it may reassess this risk after the 2014 Filing Season.

Opportunities exist to increase the efficiency and effectiveness of the IRS's use of the information reported in verifying compliance with the Affordable Care Act

The IRS plans to use the information from Provisions 1502, 1514, and 9010 to cross-verify compliance with various tax provisions the IRS is responsible for administering. The IRS has developed a separate implementation plan for each of the information reporting provisions and has assigned responsibility for implementation to different IRS functions. Figure 3 shows the IRS functional area responsible for implementing the specific provisions.

Figure 3: IRS Functional Areas Responsible for
Implementing Key Information Reporting Provisions

Affordable Care Act Provision	IRS Function
1502	Affordable Care Act Office
1514	Affordable Care Act Office
9002	Small Business/Self-Employed Division
9010	Large Business and International Division

Source: IRS Affordable Care Act Office.

However, creating separate implementation plans and assigning responsibility to different IRS offices may result in the IRS not evaluating these provisions collectively to ensure that it is requesting all the information needed to effectively verify employer, insurance provider, and individual compliance with the Affordable Care Act. For example, requiring employers to provide the name of their employee health insurance plan provider as part of Provision 1514 and the amount of health insurance premiums associated with individuals covered under a qualified health plan as part of Provision 1502 would improve the IRS's ability to ensure that all health insurance providers are submitting information returns under Provision 9010 and are, therefore, accurately assessed the annual fee.

However, the draft information return for Provision 1514 does not require employers to provide the name of their employee health insurance plan provider, and the draft information return for Provision 1502 does not require insurers to provide the amount of premiums written for employees covered by a qualified health plan.

Figure 4 provides an outline of the information currently required by each reporting provision and additional information that may improve the IRS's ability to ensure compliance.

Figure 4: Information Currently Required to Be Reported to the IRS and Additional Information That Could Improve the IRS's Ability to Ensure Compliance With Affordable Care Act Provisions

Provision	Reporting Party	Information Required to Be Reported	Additional Information That if Requested May Improve Ability to Ensure Compliance With Provisions
1502	Health insurance providers.	Names of the individuals obtaining health coverage, dates of health coverage, and whether the health coverage is a qualified health plan offered through an Exchange.	Total premiums written associated with qualified coverage provided by the insurer.
1514	Employers with more than 50 full-time equivalents in the previous year.	Whether the company offers its employees and their dependents the opportunity to enroll in minimum essential health care coverage, the period an employee must wait to become enrolled, and information regarding those employees who are enrolled in such coverage. The employer must also provide full-time employees a copy of the information return it provides to the IRS.	Name of the insurance provider used by the employer to provide group health coverage.
9002	Employers with more than 250 Forms W-2 in the previous year.	The total dollar value of health insurance coverage sponsored by the employer on each employee's annual Form W-2.	No additional information needed.
9010	Health insurance providers.	A premiums report that includes the covered entity's net premiums written during the fee year.	No additional information needed.

Source: TIGTA analysis of Provisions 1502, 1514, 9002, and 9010 of the Affordable Care Act.

Figure 5 shows how the information received from the four information reporting provisions can be used collectively to verify compliance with other tax provisions in the Affordable Care Act.

Figure 5: Use of Information
From Provisions 1502, 1514, 9002, and 9010

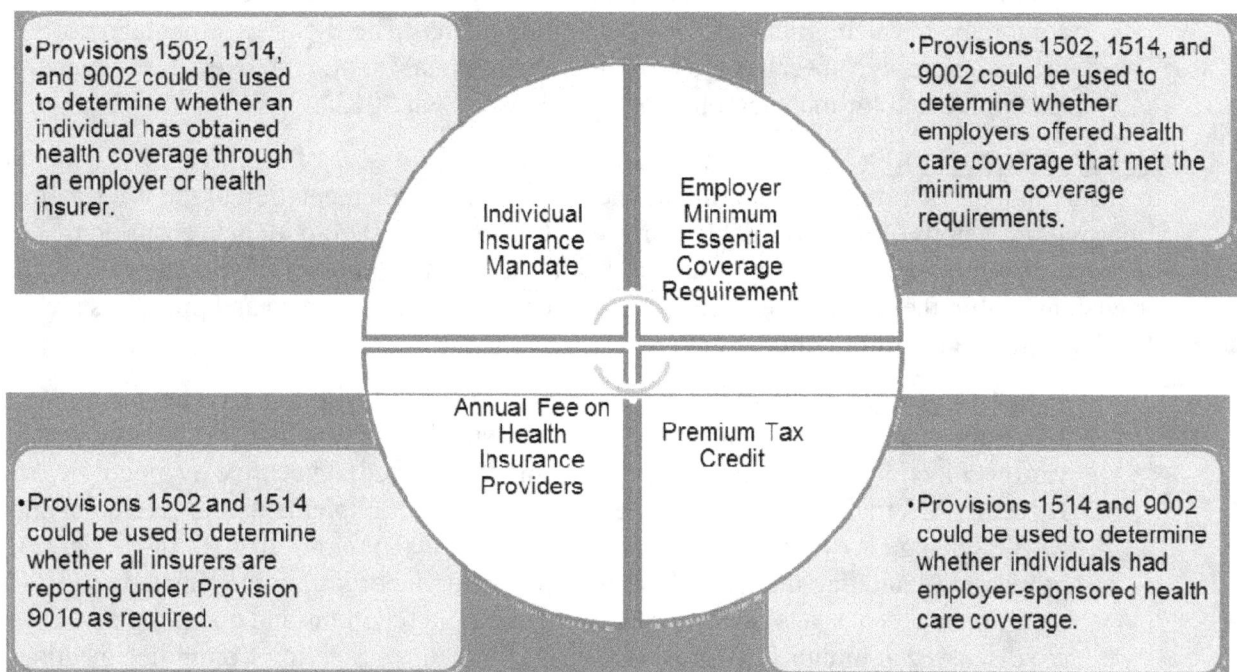

Source: *TIGTA analysis of Provisions 1502, 1514, 9002, and 9010 of the Affordable Care Act.*

Tax provisions included in the Affordable Care Act represent the largest set of tax law changes the IRS has had to implement in more than 20 years. Many of the tax provisions are interrelated. As such, the IRS must ensure that its planning efforts identify the relationships among the various tax and information reporting provisions. The IRS must then ensure that all the information needed to accurately and efficiently administer these provisions is provided either by employers, insurers, or taxpayers. By doing so, the IRS can significantly improve its ability to manage the burden placed on employers, insurers, and taxpayers who must comply with the various Affordable Care Act requirements as well as improve its ability to accurately administer Affordable Care Act fees, penalties, and tax credits.

Recommendations

The Deputy Commissioner for Services and Enforcement should:

Recommendation 1: Update the Provision 9002 implementation plan to identify the actions needed to verify that employers are accurately reporting the aggregate cost of health insurance coverage provided to an employee.

Management's Response: IRS management agreed with this recommendation. During TIGTA's audit fieldwork, the IRS was in the process of updating the Compliance Plan for Provision 9002. The Compliance Plan includes steps to verify reporting compliance, which is standard practice during audits. The IRS's prior plan did not include these steps because the reporting was optional for all employers for Calendar Year 2011 and for many employers for Calendar Year 2012.

Recommendation 2: Evaluate the planning efforts for Provisions 1502, 1514, 9002, and 9010 to ensure that all IRS functions coordinate the planning for implementation of the information reporting provisions of the Affordable Care Act. Coordination should include ensuring that all information necessary to maximize the IRS's ability to verify compliance with other tax-related provisions within the Affordable Care Act is requested from third parties and processes are developed to use the information effectively.

Management's Response: IRS management agreed with this recommendation. While management responsibility for the provisions TIGTA audited was placed in various functions (depending on the stakeholder impacted), executive oversight by the Director, Affordable Care Act Office, and the Director, Implementation Oversight and Non-Exchange Provisions, ensures that the overall planning for all Affordable Care Act provisions, including the ones affecting information reporting, is coordinated. Additionally, issues and decisions affecting multiple functions and operating divisions are discussed at monthly Affordable Care Act Executive Steering Committee meetings and during the biweekly Affordable Care Act Coordinating Committee meetings.

Appendix I

Detailed Objective, Scope, and Methodology

Our overall objective was to determine whether the IRS is effectively implementing select Affordable Care Act[1] reporting requirements. To accomplish this objective, we:

I.   Evaluated whether the IRS has identified and scheduled actions necessary to implement Affordable Care Act Provisions 1502, 1514, 9002, and 9010.

   A. Determined whether the IRS has identified all actions necessary to implement the provisions and determined whether the IRS will complete actions timely. We did this by contacting responsible parties in the Affordable Care Act Office to discuss what steps have been taken to identify the actions needed to implement the selected Affordable Care Act provisions.

   1. Determined whether the selected provisions require revisions or development of new forms, schedules, instructions, and publications.

   2. Determined whether the selected provisions would require IRS employees to receive early and/or additional training to ensure that all outside inquiries receive the proper response.

   3. Determined whether the IRS included an evaluation of the risk of fraud associated with the implementation of the selected provisions and included the actions necessary to address that risk in its implementation plan.

   B. Assessed the adequacy of the IRS's plans to obtain and use the information returns required to be provided to the IRS.

   1. Reviewed the reporting requirements created by the Affordable Care Act for the selected provisions to identify what information will be required to be reported and the taxpayers affected by the reporting requirements.

   2. Determined whether new processes are required to be developed to receive and use the reporting information provided to the IRS.

   3. Identified steps taken – either planned or completed – to update IRS processes and systems to enable taxpayers to submit required information and for the IRS to receive and use it.

---

[1] The Patient Protection and Affordable Care Act of 2010, Pub. L. No. 111-148, 124 Stat. 119 (2010) (codified as amended in scattered sections of the U.S. Code), as amended by the Health Care and Education Reconciliation Act of 2010, Pub. L. No. 111-152, 124 Stat. 1029.

II.   Evaluated whether guidance developed and/or issued for the selected reporting provisions was accurate.

    A. Identified all draft and published guidance produced by the IRS relating to the selected provisions.

    B. Assessed whether guidance provided to taxpayers and practitioners accurately reflects the requirements promulgated by the Affordable Care Act.

Internal controls methodology

Internal controls relate to management's plans, methods, and procedures used to meet their mission, goals, and objectives. Internal controls include the processes and procedures for planning, organizing, directing, and controlling program operations. They include the systems for measuring, reporting, and monitoring program performance. We determined the following internal controls were relevant to our audit objective: the controls in place to ensure that the IRS is meeting implementation dates for the Affordable Care Act reporting provisions. We evaluated the controls by reviewing the planning process used to implement Provisions 1502, 1514, 9002, and 9010 of the Affordable Care Act.

Appendix II

Major Contributors to This Report

Russell P. Martin, Acting Inspector General for Audit (Returns Processing and Account Services)
Augusta R. Cook, Acting Inspector General for Audit (Compliance and Enforcement Operations)
Deann Baiza, Director
Sharla Robinson, Audit Manager
Linna K Hung, Lead Auditor
Linda L Bryant, Senior Auditor
Denise Gladson, Auditor

Appendix III

Report Distribution List

Acting Commissioner C
Office of the Commissioner – Attn: Chief of Staff C
Commissioner, Large Business and International Division SE:LB
Commissioner, Small Business/Self-Employed Division SE:S
Director, Affordable Care Act Office SE:ACA
Director, Compliance Strategy and Policy, Affordable Care Act Office SE:ACA
Director, Filing and Premium Tax Credit Strategy, Affordable Care Act Office SE:ACA
Director, Pre-Filing and Technical Guidance, Large Business and International Division
SE:LB:PFTG
Director, Specialty Programs, Small Business/Self-Employed Division SE:S:SP
Chief Counsel CC
National Taxpayer Advocate TA
Director, Office of Legislative Affairs CL:LA
Director, Office of Program Evaluation and Risk Analysis RAS:O
Office of Internal Control OS:CFO:CPIC:IC
Audit Liaison: Affordable Care Act Office SE:ACA

Appendix IV

Glossary of Terms

Term	Definition
Calendar Year	The 12-consecutive-month period ending on December 31.
Filing Season	A 12-consecutive-month period ending on the last day of any month, except December. The Federal Government's fiscal year begins on October 1 and ends on September 30.
Full-Time Equivalent	A measure of labor hours in which one full-time equivalent is equal to eight hours multiplied by the number of compensable days in a particular fiscal year.
Health Insurance Exchange	A Health Insurance Exchange is a set of State-regulated and standardized health care plans from which individuals may purchase health insurance.
Individual Health Insurance Mandate	Individuals who do not obtain health insurance will be subject to a penalty. The individual health insurance mandate requires individuals to maintain minimum essential health insurance coverage.
Information Return	A tax document that businesses are required to file to report certain business transactions to the IRS.
Premium Tax Credit	A refundable and advanceable credit to assist individuals in purchasing affordable health insurance.
Tax Year	The 12-month period for which tax is calculated. For most individual taxpayers, the tax year is synonymous with the calendar year.
Webinar	A seminar or other presentation that takes place on the Internet that allows participants in different locations to see the presenters and ask questions.

Appendix V

Management's Response to the Draft Report

MAR 1 8 2013

MEMORANDUM FOR ACTING DEPUTY INSPECTOR GENERAL FOR AUDIT

FROM: Sarah Hall Ingram *Sarah Hall Ingram*
               Director, Affordable Care Act Office

SUBJECT: Draft Audit Report – Affordable Care Act: Implementation of Key
               Information Reporting Provisions – Audit # 201240322
               (e-trak #2013-39858)

Thank you for the opportunity to review and respond to the subject draft audit report.

I am pleased that your report acknowledges the progress IRS has made in implementing the information reporting requirements relating to Provisions 1502, 1514, 9002 and 9010 of the Affordable Care Act. As the report notes, we have identified the information employers and insurers are required to provide for each of the provisions you audited and we have developed draft forms that will be used to report this information. Our current efforts continue to evolve as regulations are finalized and will focus on process development, outreach communications and employee training.

The IRS agrees with the two recommendations contained in the report and has already taken appropriate action, as outlined in the attachment. If you have any questions, please contact me at (202) 622-6992 or Frederick W. Schindler, Director, Implementation Oversight and Non-Exchange Provisions at (202) 283-7650.

Attachment

Attachment

Draft Audit Report - Affordable Care Act: Implementation of Key Information Reporting Provisions
(Audit 201240322) (e-trak# **2013-39858**)

RECOMMENDATION #1:

The Deputy Commissioner for Services and Enforcement should update the Provision 9002
implementation plan to verify that employers are accurately reporting the aggregate cost of health
insurance coverage provided to an employee.

CORRECTIVE ACTION #1: We agree with this recommendation. During TIGTA's audit fieldwork,
IRS was in the process of updating the Compliance Plan for Provision 9002. The Compliance Plan
includes steps to verify reporting compliance, which is standard practice during package audits. Our prior
plan did not include these steps because the reporting was optional for all employers in 2011 and for
many employers for 2012.

IMPLEMENTATION DATE: Completed

RESPONSIBLE OFFICIAL: Director, Examination Policy, Small Business/Self-Employed Division

CORRECTIVE ACTION MONITORING PLAN: N/A.

RECOMMENDATION #2:

The Deputy Commissioner for Services and Enforcement should evaluate the planning efforts for
Provision 1502, 1514, 9002 and 9010 to ensure that all IRS functions coordinate the planning for
implementation of the information reporting provisions of the Affordable Care Act. Coordination should
include ensuring that all information necessary to maximize the IRS's ability to verify compliance with
other tax-related provisions within the Affordable Care Act is requested from third parties and processes
are developed to use the information effectively.

CORRECTIVE ACTION #2: We agree with this recommendation. While management responsibility
for the provisions TIGTA audited was placed in various functions (depending on the stakeholder
impacted), executive oversight by the Director, ACA Office and the Director, Implementation Oversight
and Non-Exchange Provisions ensures that the overall planning for all ACA provisions, including the
ones impacting information reporting, is coordinated. Additionally, issues and decisions impacting
multiple functions and operating divisions are discussed at the monthly ACA Executive Steering
Committee meeting and during the biweekly ACA Coordinating Committee meetings.

IMPLEMENTATION DATE: Completed/Ongoing

RESPONSIBLE OFFICIAL: Director, Affordable Care Act Office

CORRECTIVE ACTION MONITORING PLAN: N/A.

Page Intentionally Left Blank

Page Intentionally Left Blank

Page Intentionally Left Blank

Page Intentionally Left Blank

Page Intentionally Left Blank

www.ingramcontent.com/pod-product-compliance
Lightning Source LLC
Chambersburg PA
CBHW081421170526
45166CB00010B/3425